An Inspirational Journey Through Brain Surgery and Beyond!

By Mary Ann Windham

About the author:

From the earliest moment I can recall, I was fascinated by the seven different personalities (I am the youngest of seven children) that grew from our one set of parents. Though we shared the same parents who held the same expectations for all of us, governed us by the same rules, and disciplined us with the same consequences, we all saw life, and each other, differently. The discovery of each new difference between the nine of us (parents included) amazed me from the start and has continued to grow as the years unfolded.

Since then, and maybe because of that, I have been intrigued by the stories other's share with me. Stories of their own life experiences, whether similar to my own or not.

It is my belief, that in sharing our life stories we might help shed light, give hope, educate, or simply open the minds and hearts of others in new ways. In giving of ourselves, we ultimately give light to our own purpose for having journeyed through that which we have and inspire others in their own journey along the way.

I hope in sharing my most recent adventure....I might inspire some of you to embrace your own life challenges (health or otherwise) in a new way. Or, that in sharing my story you might be inspired to see things, either in your own life or in the life of someone you know, differently. But most of all, I hope that it inspires all of you to hold onto your faith and to be there for one another, as you will read....many in our little community did for us.

A short time ago, I was blessed to have been found to have a brain aneurysm. This is my story of our life's interruption and the journey we have traveled since:

Definitions to help you:

Magnetic Resonance Imaging (MRI):
is a non-invasive way to take pictures of the body using powerful magnets and radio waves.

Magnetic Resonance Angiography (MRA):
is an MRI exam of the blood vessels, considered non-invasive.

Computed Tomography Imaging also known as a CT scan (or CAT scan):
is a particular type of x-ray that uses multiple x-ray beams at different angles to build up a cross section of the body's organs and tissues.

Arteriography:
is test that uses x-rays and a special dye to see inside the arteries. It can be used to see arteries in the heart, brain, kidney, and many other parts of the body.

Arteriogram:
is a special type of x-ray picture to see the blood vessels called arteries.

Table of Contents:

Chapter 1 - How it was found

Chapter 2 - Moving forward through the diagnosis

Chapter 3 - Sharing the secret

Chapter 4 - The procedure I would be awake through

Chapter 5 - Results move us forward on a more defined path

Chapter 6 - News of the solution shared

Chapter 7 - The surgery

Chapter 8 - Recovery begins

Chapter 9 - The tape!

Chapter 10 - The removal of the staples that lined my face

Chapter 11 - Now let's move back toward normal life…slowly!

Table of Contents Continued:

Chapter 12 – The headaches

Chapter 13 – Meeting "Mr. Spaz"

Chapter 14 - Four months post-surgery

Chapter 15 – By the end of summer

Chapter 16 – Five Years Post Surgery

Chapter 17 – The reflection collection

How it was found

I was just over forty six years old when during a visit with one of my older siblings (I am the youngest child, so they're all older…LOL) she shared with me her life's journey concerning a hearing issue.

As soon as she mentioned it I recalled, somewhere from the back of my mind, her having some issue with this growing up. However, nothing really stuck out about the details of her loss, so at first I regretted not recalling more. Although, as she said, for years she compensated and worked around it, learning to adapt and not draw attention to it, which helped the rest of us not focus on it as well. In the past few years we have been separated geographically, only seeing each other on holidays or family weddings. We exchanged the occasional letters to share our child's photo, or special accomplishment. Which is again why it just did not stand out to me at the time.

It was not until *this* visit that we have had much time to reconnect and share who we had become. It was then she had time to speak to me about how much more challenging her life had become in dealing with the increasing hearing loss over the last few years.

She told me about how much more difficult it had become, especially in her business life, to guess at the missing words, piece together what she did hear, and then follow along in conversations. Even as an astute listener, her efforts had become focused on trying to decide, quickly, which person spoke the most important part of the conversation, so she could position herself to see their lips best. She shared how challenging it had grown to be if someone was not positioned just right or if they spoke too fast, I imagined her struggle and was struck by her openly honest sharing, and felt happy to have this time to reconnect.

It was not until I returned home I realized how much it all stuck with me. Over and over in my head I heard her describing how now, later in life, her disability had become a bigger issue and created much more of a challenge - the lip reading and the positioning herself, especially the challenge in crowds. Soon I could no longer escape the similarities to my own experiences; I <u>too</u> had learned and become dependent on lip reading well and on positioning myself right, in an effort to stay engaged with people. I <u>too</u> had accepted missing out on parts of conversations as "normal and natural" and it had all come to play a role in my own way of life as well. Quickly, I became increasingly aware of how often I burdened conversations with (to my mother's disgust, I am sure) "Huh?", "What?", or an "Excuse me?" I began to realize how hard I worked at positioning myself to see others lips in crowded places, in order to figure out what they were saying. I began to realize how often I just chose to dropout of conversations because I could not hear well enough to keep up.

Until one day my concerns and curiosity (thanks to her sharing her own journey) grew so much that it led me to make an appointment with my own doctor. Little did I realize then, that was only the beginning of my most recent life's journey.

I started with a visit to our local hearing specialist (at the advice of my family doctor) to have my hearing evaluated. I recall thinking to myself… "Oh its age, or maybe selective hearing". That's what we all once thought my father's hearing issue was. Being a father with five girls and only two boys…who would not shut out female voices, right? However, ironically my father was found later to have a hearing disability that required hearing aids. So, I went through the process....made my appointment, was tested and evaluated, and was asked to return for follow up results in two weeks. Ugh, I hate that part…*the waiting*! But it had to be done, so I scheduled the return appointment.

As always, I scheduled the appointment just prior to going to work one day. Why not? I also thought little of going alone, since I was confident it was something simple... no big deal, right? Boy was I wrong! But let's not get ahead of ourselves.

Two weeks later, I returned for my follow up appointment and it turned out that I had a hearing loss in *each* ear and that loss had an added problem. My loss was not a balanced loss from ear to ear, as in the case of most. Mine just had to be different! My loss was present, but vastly different in each ear. "But not to worry…you can correct that with a pair of hearing aids! Of course most insurance policies do **not** cover hearing aids and the best ones for you would be mid-range ones, costing <u>only</u> 4000 dollars!"

Beyond the cost of hearing aids there would be time for follow ups, adjustments, re-adjustments, re-programming, etc, etc.

Ever think we should get paid or a credit against their bill, for the time it takes for them to get back to us? Or one for the length of our time it takes for them to attend to our issue? Is not our time also important, we are the ones who spend that time suffering, not them! Maybe if they had to pay us or give us a credit, they would be quicker about tending to us and not seem to think they have the rest of our lives to do so. And what about the wasted time and money spent on inconclusive test? Ever think you should have to pay for those test that did not do any good? You know, those tests that were run just for the sake of process? Not me!

Anyway... I was shell shocked and I am not sure what shocked me more, the dual hearing issue or the cost of dual hearing aids, not covered by my insurance. We have to hear, don't we? It's not like I chose to be this way, or that I did anything that caused it purposefully or neglectfully! However, there was nothing I could do about that now.... and I still had to go to work from here! I worked with the public and had an eight hour day ahead of me. What a day this was going to be!

Although, of course before going on to work I took time out to call my husband along the way. I announced the findings and shared the shock, and forewarned him of the expense that lie ahead of us. I called also hoping I could offer him time to think it over (and have his own truthful reactions in peace) before I arrived home at the end of my work day.

Poor thing, he was as shocked as I was, but…he was also sweetly supportive. He merely reassured me over and over that it would be fine and we would do whatever we needed to do. I am so blessed to have him by my side! Before I knew it, we were on the same page...adjust, adapt, accept, and move through it (because, truly, was there any other choice?). I'd been through worse things in my life. It is just a part of life…I convinced myself.

Moving forward through the diagnosis

Soon, the process of the hearing aids and their adjustments, visits and re-visits began. During one of those many visits the hearing specialist recommended I see an ENT (ear, nose and throat specialist) for my unusual loss. Although hearing aids were the answer, we still needed to figure out the cause. Something we later found he should have done after my original visit/findings, however for reasons of his own (those we do not know); he waited 'til now.

So off to yet another doctor for more tests.

I scheduled the ENT appointment, this time taking the day off and my husband along with me. I had learned from the previous appointment to be more prepared for anything…or so I thought. The ENT did his routine blood work, exam, and expressed his own curiosity in my unusual loss and then sent us for an MRI (just for a closer look inside) and told us again…. "See you in two weeks!" Did I tell you I hate that part? I was not sure if his intrigue was a good thing or not, but we were on a roll now and committed to finding answers.

Two weeks later, we went back for answers to what caused the hearing problem that seemed so "unique", even though by this time it was being corrected with hearing aids.

What we received was a two page report informing us that there was more than a hearing loss to worry about. The report showed there were several issues going on…not all hearing related. In fact...he had no real explanation for the hearing issue itself, but had a more important issue that needed to be addressed <u>immediately</u>.

Most importantly, I had what was believed to be an aneurysm on my carotid artery. "That's in my brain (I heard myself say…and then scream over and over inside my head)!" My heart stopped and my mind panicked, as it tried to absorb the words that followed…but am sure I missed most of. I recall my mind going blank...and the sensation of walking off into a fog of self-preservation, holding onto the peace I have often found in my faith at times like these. Thank goodness my husband was there to absorb the rest of the doctor's comments and knew to ask for copies of the report for a closer look once we would arrive home.

In the meantime, the ENT scheduled me to see the local neurologist and ordered yet another test, an MRA (**Magnetic Resonance Angiography**). Upon setting up the appointment the neurologist's office told the ENT's staff that it would be several weeks before I could get in. Which is when he insisted that the neurologist call him immediately (on his personal cell phone) to make other arrangements. We were impressed to find that he cared enough about us to take *this* step, but then too, worried about the urgency of it all….and PANIC set in! "That is not something most doctors do…was there something more to it?" They tried to assure us that it was merely something they felt strongly was not to be put off as a trivial issue, not because there was anything to be overly concerned with. While we tried to accept that as reassuring….our minds were too focused on the priority he placed on my case to accept that that was all it was.

We left the ENT's office that day going through the motions…we went immediately to the local hospital, signed in, had the test and were immediately given a copy of the MRA on CD (impressed to find we could have such a thing and so quickly).

A couple of days later, we found ourselves in the neurologist's office going through a battery of tests (stand on one foot, close your eyes and touch your nose, repeat back this list of things, who's the president….). Then he gave us his opinion of what he saw on the MRA. To him the results showed the aneurysm, but the results appeared inconclusive as to its size, exact placement and shape. The size, shape and placement are pieces of information that were needed to determine what solution followed. From what he could see the aneurysm was pressing on the optic nerve in my left eye (nothing to do with my hearing issue) so the first thing we needed to do is have a field of vision test to check how my vision might be affected by the aneurysm or by the surgery to fix it! After that, a more conclusive test would be needed to determine the size, shape and placement to know how we would proceed from here.

So began yet <u>another</u> roller coaster with yet <u>another</u> set of doctors, none of which were in the same offices, or even nearby! They were not even in the same small town (of course).

That same day, we headed to our family eye doctor, where he would perform the field of vision test. This test was performed to see the entire area (field) of how well each of my eyes could see independently. I placed my face into a large white machine with one central red focal point, while the attendant ran me through a series of tiny scattered lights. To each tiny light I saw (or thought I saw) I would record it by pressing a remote she placed in my hand. The test was first performed on my left eye and then my right for comparison. It was painless as well as quick and we were given an immediate copy of the results (yeah!). To our amazement, and the amazement of my doctors, there was little damage found at all!

      Days after leaving the neurologist's office and the eye doctor, I was scheduled to see a neurosurgeon! This was huge! So in the time between my field of vision appointment and the appointment with the neurosurgeon we contacted my sister (who not only had the hearing issue, but also has a medical background) and got online to gather information. We were determined to be as prepared as we could be to understand what he might tell us about what lie ahead. Plus, my husband wanted to be informed of this surgeon's skills, abilities and reputation (isn't he the greatest?).

Once online, we were very pleased to find my neurosurgeon was not <u>only</u> at the top of his class in brain related aneurysm surgeries, he was also the top of his class in educating other to do the same. We were both breathing a sigh of relief at that point, of course. Thank God for small blessings…each and every one!

The appointment with the neurosurgeon began with the same silly test of balance, mental capability and common probing questions as those ran at the neurologist's office. The silly tests were then followed by a small conversation to explain what an aneurysm was, how many ways patients can get one, and how dangerous it would be to leave it unattended.

Aneurysms can be painful, but not always create pain (like mine). Some can exist for quite some time and be undetected (like mine, until now), and some can rupture before they are found. Any brain aneurysm that ruptures causes damage to the surrounding area and are often terminal, because of the damage they do in the first

<u>four</u> hours before diagnosis and treatment comes into play.

They can be hereditary (although no one that I know of in my family has had one), you can get one from smoking (I was a light smoker for years until about three years ago), you can get one from a severe injury (I had fallen, as a toddler, from high up on a flight of stairs, landing on a tile floor around the same area of my head) and the origin of some are unexplained.

In his opinion there was no way to tell how long I had had mine or what specifically caused it for sure. However, the one thing he could do was run <u>another</u> test to see more clearly its exact size and shape, as well as where it was specifically located. This information, we learned, was needed "*if we chose to address the aneurysm*", because it would help him determine which of the two procedures would be available to me from here. So my appointment was followed with an immediate on-site CAT scan (Computed Tomography Imaging) with contrast that was again quick and painless. And yes, to get the results….. another "we'll see you back in two weeks for results!" UGH!!!! However, this one was followed with, "by the way...don't stress yourself over this in the meantime...it is not good for your condition." Yeah right!

The two possible options for my treatment, *"should we choose to address it"*, were to have a "coiling procedure" or a "clipping procedure".

In the coiling procedure, they go in through the groin and up the artery to the brain, to place small metal coils or springs inside the aneurysm. The coils fill the aneurysm to prevent the pressure of blood flow from causing it to rupture leading to a stroke and further damage. This process would then require follow ups yearly, for the rest of my life, to make sure the coils stayed in place and did not compress. If that were to happen the process would need to be repeated again and again, as many times as necessary.

The clipping procedure required major surgery, going through the scalp, the facial muscles, inside the skull, and into the affected area of the brain, to place a small titanium clip across the neck of the aneurysm. This clip would close off the blood flow, preventing it from ever rupturing. In some cases (like mine, of course) an additional entry into the neck is also required. The incision here is to reach the artery in order to place a temporary clamp, closing off the blood flow, so that the aneurysm is held still while the titanium clip can be put securely in place. Then the clamp in the neck is released and incision closed with both internal stitches and external taping (you'll read more about this later). The clipping process would then require some surgical follow up the first few months and one a year later. But then we would be done with it for the rest of my life! Hum...which would I prefer???

Of course, doing either procedure could also cause the aneurysm to rupture (possibly causing stroke or worse).

We returned for our follow up, after what seemed like years of living each day on edge waiting and hoping it did not explode, to find yet another test would need to be done before the decision could be made.

My "unique" (as doctors now repeatedly referred to it) aneurysm had yet another twist. The bone was in the way of visualizing it no matter what angle or depth they took the pictures from, so a procedure called a carotid arteriogram (a special type of x-ray picture to see the blood vessels in your neck that carry blood to the brain) would now have to be done in order to be conclusive of the path we should take. For this procedure, I would have to be awake, even though it was a surgical procedure. Yikes!

Sharing the secret

Up to this point we had not told our families or friends anything about my condition. We thought to ourselves, it was because we felt we had not yet had enough detail about what we were dealing with and what we would be facing to answer any questions comfortably. This was partly true. In reality, I can say now, we also needed that time to figure out how we would rest with it ourselves and until we did there seemed little point in sharing it. Besides in my family, once you share it with one person the "family grapevine" starts and conversations fly, and as I said...we did not have all the answers yet.

As things were more confirmed and the tests had become more involved ……it was time to tell, time to accept its realness and….time to take that first committed (no turning back) step into the process.

Now came the question...how do we share it and with whom do we start?

The answer to the second part of that question seemed the easiest; we would start with my mother and our children. We would start with those who lived closest to us, who could not only be supportive and encouraging, but also there in the hours of need that lie ahead. They were the ones that would (could) be at our sides if we found ourselves in need of extra hands for any issue that might arise.

What did not seem so obvious is *how* we would tell them. And yet, as many things had gone so far, the moment we needed the answer it seemed odd how in alignment the world was to supply us with exactly that.

Now, I know television is controversial with many and that many shows involve stories about characters acting a part. However, I also know many times those parts are written in scripts designed by people who are often basing them off of real life stories they know, or stories they have heard of. So just follow me when I say....it was strange how even in the moments we tried to escape the ordeal and watch television, there it was....another show about what we were facing. There was someone either facing the same thing, or caring for someone who was, or someone who had. Each show offered examples of how someone else had chosen to travel through the journey, similar to mine. Of course, it was partly to do with the fact that some of our favorite shows were things like "Grey's Anatomy", "House" and "NCIS".

The shows offered options on how to cope and allowed us time to explore, talk and share our feelings in a more comfortable way. It allowed us time to feel okay with whatever passing thought or feeling we had…at least for moments at a time and then set it aside for a while.

However, soon without really discussing it in great detail, we decided, both independently and jointly, to face the whole situation with humor. Yes, humor! We are not people who live for real drama, so this just seemed fitting!

In our first weeks of discovery, tests, and appointments, my husband and I had already chosen to face things amongst ourselves with humor, without really even discussing it. It just seemed the easiest when running from doctor to doctor, waiting for tests, waiting for the results, waiting to get their opinions and hoping the aneurysm would not rupture in the meantime. It was the humor that kept us going. It is part of who my husband *is* and one of the parts of him I fell in love with, so many years ago.

You would be surprised how taking a humorous view on difficult things can really seem to make them so much lighter to carry. And while others are left wondering if you have simply lost your mind, joking about something so serious, you will find yourself not only enlightened, but empowered with how inspiring you can be to them or them to you.

Now I know, you are saying... you have got to be kidding! And those that know me really must have thought I had lost my mind, knowing I once suffered from anxiety attacks that were so bad I was house bound for quite some time. But I am telling you... humor is a much better way of life. Really what other choice did we have? It was that or crumble! And as fast as things were moving....crumbling just did not seem like something we had time for. I was not going back to life filled with anxiety!

Of course inside ourselves, we had our moments of fear, doubt, and overwhelming panic from time to time. We are human!

However, we also have our faith and through that, it just seemed instinctive to us both now, to hold strong to that inner faith that has always been there to offer us peace of mind in times of great challenge. And in doing so....the humor just came easily. Even I was amazed at how quickly it made the tough times that much more comfortable to carry (at least in appearance). I think being "upbeat" for each other, as well as those who love us, was our way of making it easier on everyone….them, as well as ourselves.

For me, I also wanted to protect the time we had left (short or long). I hoped that as things went along, I could hold onto that strength, that faith and humor had given me and allow me to be an inspiration to those around me. I love being an inspiration to others: to me….what better gift could I give? And should the plan for me not be that things went as I hoped.....I wanted to be remembered in that way. I wanted those left behind to have fun memories of me to share with each other, in hopes that it would bring them closer together in a tough time. Learning this from "My Sweetie" has been one of the many valuable gifts he has given me....and now, one I could pass along to our children too.

Anyway…..

We walked through the next weeks disclosing our secret, first to my mother and our children. Then disclosing it to our family members, friends, coworkers, slowly, absorbing quickly the power and strength from their prayers and encouragement. Holding on to their love and support, and laughing our way through each day that passed. You would be surprised how many jokes you can make and how much fun you can have with a brain aneurysm when it is all your own.

Before we knew it…we were loved and supported by not only our friends, family, and co-workers, but also by what seemed like everyone in our new quaint little home town and beyond! It was amazing! Each new day gave me more hope and confidence that I…that WE would come through this….. JUST FINE! The love and laughter was working!

*The procedure
I would be awake through*

The carotid arteriogram, ordered by the neurosurgeon, was quite interesting.

We arrived early that November morning and were taken straight to the pre-op room where staff came in (one by one), introducing themselves, beginning their lists of questions and tasks to perform. Even my neurosurgeon arrived and checked in (in a timely fashion, of course) just to be on standby, should something go awry during the procedure (since this procedure can cause the aneurysm to rupture) and to take an immediate look at the results.

Par for course (for me), the nurses had to make several attempts before a properly working IV could be run. However, soon enough, we were under way and ready…..to *wait* for the radiologist to arrive (he was not so timely). Once he did arrive, I was wheeled into a nearby surgical room, where I was introduced to that staff, prepped further, and *waited* yet again for the radiologist to arrive, this time much more anxiously.

Once he came into the room, he briefly explained what lie ahead, called for a sedative to help me relax and began. He immediately numbed my groin (femoral artery) with a simple solution and cut a pencil tip eraser size hole, of which I felt little to nothing, it was weird. He then inserted a catheter (thin tube) into the hole and up into the carotid artery…. up and across my entire body into the carotid artery in my neck and into my brain! Thank goodness I was given that medication to help me relax and remain comfortable. Not that it was painful, but it was definitely weird to think they were making this piece of tubing travel through my body guided by a video camera and just slightly unsettling!

From here it was my job to remain very still and follow the doctor's direction each time he asked me to close my eyes, take a deep breath and hold it while counting to 30, slowly, then *wait*…. while he injected the iodine dye (contrast material) through the tube and into the affected area of my brain (yikes). As I did my job each time, *waited* for the BURNING of the dye in my brain to start, lasting 30 seconds (seemed like longer while it was burning) and then ease off. It made me think this must have been a bit like what Frankenstein felt in the lab (poor man).

I could feel the dye burn like acid and see it light up the vessels and arteries from behind my closed eyelids with the whitest of white color like I had never seen before. Thank goodness each time it only lasted 30 seconds. However, it was done, probably twelve times! Each time the dye was injected, the X-ray machine moved about me to every possible angle. It had to be done like this because the more pictures meant better detail and the more I lay still, the clearer those pictures would be.

After each round of dye injections and x-rays taken, I was permitted to open my eyes (and breathe) again. Each time I opened my eyes I could look up and see the four large monitors placed at my side. It was truly fascinating, albeit frightening, to realize I was looking at my own brain and so was everyone else! And some people, growing up, thought I did not have a brain...LOL.

Once the many pictures were taken, to the radiologist satisfaction, (and quickly approved by the neurosurgeon, who stopped by) the catheter could be removed from my artery.

But of course, the fun did not end there....this is when one of the staff was assigned to apply pressure on the hole cut in my artery at the groin area. Extreme pressure, that is, for twenty minutes, as hard as the left-behind nurse could manage. Because, while it sounds easy, clotting off the open main artery was a matter of life and death! And to make sure she did so correctly, another staff member was left there to observe her.

Once the bleeding was stopped, it was checked and covered before I was moved (wheeled, not physically moved) into a recovery room. In the recovery room I needed to continue to lay flat without raising my head or moving my leg for at least the next four hours! Or at least that was the plan.

Normally at this point, the staff would check the patient's blood pressure, heart rate, pupils, reflexes, and groin site frequently while they received IV fluids to flush out the dye, as well as offered something for the typical headache that follows....which in my case, had already begun. So....this is when they administered "this great new medicine for that typical migraine reaction called Toradol" (a non-steroidal anti-inflammatory drug) into my body. Which is when my body again took its own "UNIQUE" course (again the doctors had chosen to call it…. and I have repeated this to you NO WHERE near as much as they did to me).

When "this great new medicine" began to work in <u>MY</u> body…it sent me into a seizure like episode. My body began shaking more and more, uncontrollably, so much so that the staff had become confused as to what to do next. By the time they figured out that it was the medicine… I was also suffering from nausea, vomiting and muscular pain like never before. None of which is good for someone who is not supposed to move, I remind you.

You see my body does not like medications, especially at what doctors call "usual adult doses". If I had a nickel for every time I tried to explain this to medical staff everywhere….I would be retired with my husband and family in our own little beach house in the community of our dreams long, long ago (of which
I am not yet, unfortunately)!

After some time, the staff administered yet another drug into my IV, in hopes to control my reaction to the Toradol. It was Phenergan. Thank God for whoever invented that drug! It brought with it, almost immediate relief. However, due to the original episode I was now to remain in recovery <u>much longer</u> than the usual 4-5 hours before being permitted to go home. This was all I hoped for at this point, wanting to be back at home and work to pass the time until my final surgery.

However we were not done yet, for once again my body took another "unique" turn when the next morning (as the Phenergan wore off) the severe headache returned with the same vengeance. Within minutes I suffered such terrible headache pain that my husband and I thought that the aneurysm *must* have ruptured. We rushed to our local emergency room, two blocks from our home, only to experience yet another nightmare, which may have been funny at this point if I was not in such extreme pain. You see, we arrived at our local hospital only to find their remodeling in progress. Jack hammering filled the entire emergency room area! It took only moments, but seemed like hours, before my poor husband could get them to shut down and move elsewhere. Boy was that ER nurse wrong when she first insisted "I cannot do anything about the jackhammers." Can you believe it?

In a matter of time they quickly performed another CAT scan to insure the aneurysm had not ruptured, before deciding how they would proceed. It had not and again we thanked God and breathed a sigh of relief! The ER doctor speculated that the pain could have been related to "that great new drug, Toradol" that I had been given the day prior. However, to confirm this he needed to confer with my neurosurgeon. He had hoped to obtain first-hand information on my case before moving too far forward. Unfortunately, my neurosurgeon (as he had already told us) was out of town. At this point we informed him that the practice they had taken the day prior was to administer the Phenergan, with great results! Thank goodness he agreed to follow suit as a temporary measure. Once administered, I found that same instant relief …. he returned to trying to contact the hospital I had been in the day prior, in hopes to get me a room where my case information would be readily accessed. Unfortunately this went on for hours, so we *waited*. In the meantime my husband had left and returned with food which was a welcome sight now that I had begun to feel better and realized I had not yet eaten all day.

Hours later, we grew antsy and insisted we be permitted to go home, where I felt I could rest in peace and quiet. However, the ER staff did not agree, though it would still be hours before a room would become available at the other hospital (they too were remodeling and short of rooms). So against medical orders….we left for home and a peaceful nights sleep. By morning I was on the mend once again, slowly but surely.

Even after I returned to work a couple days later, my coordination was a bit wobbly and my sense of judgment in distance was as well. This made even simple things like pouring coffee a bit difficult! My head felt strange and the burning shots of lights continued on for quite some time, however for shorter periods each time. It was a full week later before I felt somewhat back to normal and rid of all the dye (which my neurosurgeon told me once again was "unique but not unheard of"). Now we just waited for the neurosurgeons' final decision about which surgical procedure he would allow me to have, though we hoped secretly for the clipping. We hoped he would suggest the clipping because we felt it offered greater comfort to know that the aneurysm would be fixed completely and allow us to be free to return to life as we had previously known…worry free (well, you know what I mean).

Results move us forward on a more defined path

The results of the carotid arteriogram showed my aneurysm was again a "unique" one for which we would have only one option for its repair after all. Thankfully it was the option we had already decided that we were more comfortable with.

The solution to my aneurysm issue would be the clipping procedure. It seemed my aneurysm, at this time, was presenting as 6 mm in size with a "uniquely" wide neck. It was the wide neck that brought on the need for the clipping procedure and ruled out the coiling option because the coils would not stay in place without a narrower neck to hold them in.

My aneurysm was indeed pressing on my left optic nerve, even though the previous field of vision test had shown no sign of problems as of yet. Again this made it "unique, although not unheard of". However, one of the side effects often experienced after the clipping procedure, when the aneurysm involves the optic nerve, is that there is likely be some optical nerve damage. The optical nerve doesn't like to be touched and since my aneurysm was already pressing on that nerve…it was likely it would have to be further touched. The surgeon promised he would be as un-invasive as possible.

There were risks of vision loss in my case, as well as the typical list of possible complications that come along with having this surgical procedure. The aneurysm could burst during the procedure due to the stress of the invasion to one's body during any surgery, but should it rupture…they hoped minimal damage would take place since they would be there to correct it quickly. However, any brain surgery (or major surgery) always includes the possibility of risk up to and including death. Besides, what choice was there really….sit and wait for the aneurysm to choose when it would rupture and take my life anyway? I think not!

So, while a bit overwhelming, we were happy the path was clear. We were happy because we had already decided that the one-time procedure (with the one year follow up) would be better for us than the other alternative method, which carried many more unknowns for the future.

However, having the decision made for us this way, was added assurance we were doing the right thing. Or that's the way we took it. So with the doctor's approval, a short time later….I was admitted to do just that.

News of the solution shared

In no time, my family (mine and my husband's), our friends, coworkers, and town's people had all been informed. They too had been worried and had been hoping, praying, and waiting, as had their friends, families, church members and etc. Their constant words of kindness left us feeling as if we had a whole world of prayers and support surrounding us. Feeling so loved and cared for was inspiring to us like never before. It allowed us the strength to continue to joke and have fun with our situation (you would not believe the jokes you can make up with something like this….or how many times you can play the role of the Scarecrow from the Wizard of Oz, singing…. "If I only had a brain"). Thus far we had experienced the best medical care we could hope for and were quickly moved through the process of getting to this point. We even had one of the world's best neurosurgeons to perform the procedure. We were blessed beyond our imaginations, so it was easy to leave it in the Lord's hands and know that however the journey came to be …..it was what we would be able to handle. Whether we believed it at this point or not.

No, we were not without fear, concern, and doubt…from time to time. However, with that many people on your side, that many prayers being offered in your name, and that skill level on the other end of the knife….how could you ask for more? Or doubt that it would go well? Therefore, we did not allow ourselves much time daily to dwell on what could happen otherwise.

The surgery

The night before surgery I had actually slept better than I thought I would, knowing it would soon be over and I could put the long two month process behind us. I tried to focus on the great nap that lie ahead for me, while I feared others would spend those long hours pacing and waiting…but praying for me. When I allowed myself a moment to be worried... it was as much, if not more, about what this was putting my poor husband and kids through, than what I was going through.

I went in early on a Thursday morning, just two weeks prior to the Christmas holiday. My surgery was expected to take eight hours minimum (the doctor estimated). However, mine went quickly (about 5 hours) even though the size of it was found to actually be 7 mm (rather than the 6 mm it was originally presumed to be)… and thankfully very well! This was one time when "unique" was a good thing!

In no time (for me) I woke happy to be alive, repaired and on the way to begin my long road to recovery with my husband at my side. I woke grateful for the blessings God had shown me through the doctor's wisdom, talent and knowledge…to allow me more time with my children, grandchildren, husband, family, and friends. I must have spent hours (in and out of a medicated state) being more thankful than ever before and breathing that sigh of relief over and over. Not because I had feared for myself, but because I feared for what it would bring upon those I loved had it not gone as hoped.

Now I just needed to get through the first 24 hours, those which I knew… after all major surgeries, were always the toughest.

At this point my head was wrapped in bandages and held the drain in place (the drain left to keep pressure off my brain from the surgery), and of course, an IV was running into my right hand. There was also a large bandaged area on the left side of my neck where they did have to go in and clamp the artery, in order to get it to hold still for the clip to go in place correctly and safely. I also had 5 holes in each wrist (I always seem to find they have trouble starting IV's on me) and a catheter in my bladder (common after any major surgery). I was thirsty and yes, feeling as though someone had run me over with a truck.... in a great deal of pain. But nothing like I had previously imagined, Thank God!

As expected the first twenty four hours were the worst for me (I could not be "unique" here and have it not be?). However I must admit that for me, it was mostly because of the medications.

Because it was brain surgery, they were limited to giving me Codeine to deal with the pain those first several hours. Codeine is not a mind altering drug and they need to assess your mental faculties after brain surgery to insure all is working properly. But for me Codeine created a sense that every minute hair on my body had stood on end and become a needle or pin piercing my skin. Each dose became increasingly piercing every time they gave it to me, even though it was given in smaller and smaller doses (because my husband fought their efforts to give me the adult doses that were obviously too strong for my body to handle) that came every hour.

It was the Codeine that brought on severe headaches, which brought another medication twenty minutes later, that gave me nausea, that would bring another medication twenty minutes after that to settle the nausea. So after each dose of Codeine I would have to take other medications that would help with each side effect twenty minutes apart. This cycle had to be continued all through the night until the late night/early morning staff came in.

It was with the change of staff that the discovery was made. The Codeine was also raising my blood pressure (yes, high blood pressure is not a good thing post brain/aneurysm surgery...imagine that) which was what caused the headaches and the nausea, that caused the tremors. Thank God for morning and change of staff!

Once the new staff arrived…. A blood pressure medication was administered along with new post-surgery medications that were now available for the pain and swelling. With these, the headaches settled, the nausea and tremors subsided on their own and the blood pressure was under control. I was on a much better road to recovery!

After two more days of poking, prodding, needle sticks, pain medications and neurological test, I was free to go home and leave all the heavy narcotics behind. My surgery was on Thursday morning…I went home the following Sunday afternoon, amazing what can be done these days isn't it? Ahh home! Finally, I could get some rest and care with very little drugs, from people who loved me most, as well as those who truly knew what was best for me.

Although we filled the prescriptions given upon departure....within the first 12 hours I was able to limit myself to only ibuprofen and heat packs routinely, for the pain I was left with. Not bad!

Recovery begins

My recovery plan, estimated by the doctors, was set to be a good 6-8 months out. Something that when they said it originally seemed a lot shorter then it came to be once I actually had to live it. I was bothered mostly due to the boredom I felt, being so limited as to *what* I could do more than anything. While pregnancy lasts 9 months... at least there is a cute little bundle of joy at the end, and plenty you can do in the meantime. However, at least it was winter and I was not the only one house bound and with the holidays came visitors, Thank goodness!

During the first few days at home the hardest part of my recovery was in finding things I could do working around the side effects of the swelling. The swelling inside and outside my head (and neck) interfered with my attention span, blocked parts of my vision, and drained my strength and energy level. I could not watch television (my attention span was just not that long) and I could not see well enough to read or do the many crafts I had bought, prior to surgery. I had not realized when I purchased them that my attention span would be so limited that I would not be able to do such things. I merely thought I needed to be prepared for the long road ahead.

So, I slept a lot! Some out of weakness, some from all that surgery drains from a person, some from the side effects of what little medications I still took for inflammation, as well as out of the boredom and the lack of ability to do anything else.

It was days before I was able to play some computer games and my attempts to watch television improved as my attention span lengthened gradually over time. I am not much into soap operas, so I recorded things on television at night to watch during the day. When all else failed I tried watching movies, we bought ahead of time for entertainment, and snacked…I still had my appetite, however changed it had become.

      Food now became intense at times. Everything I ate that was sweet, became way too sweet and everything salty too salty. Which I guess was not so bad, I could still eat ice cream. Ice cream was one of my favorite things as a child. I could even smell it when my parents had some after sending us kids to bed…. all the way from upstairs! Smelling ice-cream has always been my life's claim to fame with my siblings, children, and now grandchildren too.

      Something else new was my taste for ginger! Oh the holiday spices…I can still smell and taste them! I discovered my new taste for ginger when a sweet little girl, Molly, from next door brought over a holiday "get well" gift of freshly made gingerbread cookies. She and her younger brother, Dan, made me an entire plate of slightly decorated holiday characters, all made of gingerbread! Oh my gosh! I thought I had died and gone to heaven! I still crave them to this day.

But anyway…..

Thankfully, as I have said, it was holiday time so there were not only gingerbread cookies, but most of the family had come to my mother's this year too. My mother's house is not too far from our home, so it was great spending time with other people that I had not seen in a while. With lots of siblings and kids around all I had to do (thanks to my husband) was sit and enjoy the visiting.

Of course, there were also the routine follow up visits to the neurosurgeon to keep us busy too and if all else failed…there was always some light housework to help pass the time as well.

Yes, in boredom and limitations even housework can be appreciated as something to do. And through it all, my husband was incredibly supportive and helpful too. He has been patient, insightful and a real help in listening to my needs and trying to support me…. in talking more slowly (so I could register and keep up), limiting choices (to the number I could handle), and making me take care of *me!* It was important for me to begin to do things, but not overdo and that's a fine line that constantly changed during this recovery process.

The tape!

A few days after the surgery, the butterfly tape on my neck (the tape that lay across the 4 inch opening over top my artery) was supposed to show signs of coming off. This would be helped along with letting it get wet, which I did not do because that part was not made clear to me as something I should do. Instead I had spent that time protecting it from getting wet. That is until the tape began to itch and burn my neck so badly I could no longer stand it! This is when we set ourselves on a mission to get it off.

Unfortunately, the incision underneath all that tape still had healing work to do and was far too tender to let us pull on the tape much at all. It did not take much time for the real frustration to set in and when it did….. I did what I had done in years past when my girls were small and I needed advice…I called my oldest sister! She was a nurse, a mom, and my big sister…she would know what to do! I had not recalled a time, back then, when she had ever led me a stray or disappointed me by not knowing *something*

I could try, even if I did not always totally agree. So I called and slowly announced my plea and she…….. laughed!

The tape was on with a glue that I was sure was superglue! It was so gummy nothing made it budge in the slightest. The more it would not move… the more my panic set in. I think it was about power and control at this point, one of my first desperate needs to regain control over something of myself. Looking back (and even as she laughed) it was funny.

At this point I did not care if she laughed, all I cared about was …did she have some clues to get it off…and that she did, thank goodness!

First we could get it wet, I could soak it in the tub. Oh if we had only remembered knowing this, I would not have spent so much time and care not to do so prior.

Secondly, I could try something like fingernail polish remover! Oh my gosh! This sounded horrible! All I could imagine was the burn I felt in the past when I got it in a paper cut. But she said that something in polish remover (I cannot recall now what) would help break up the glue and that made sense. I was to put it on the tape (not into the incision) with a cotton swab and little by little roll the tape back and pull it free. Hey, I was desperate, so if getting it wet did not work, I was game!

Thirdly, I could try "WD40"! It *too* had something in it that would do the same thing… however, this one I decided I would take note of and hope I would not have to do. Not sure why it scared me more the fingernail polish remover (especially since I had not felt the burn of this in a cut before) but it did, so I merely noted this one for truly life and death (or close) desperation and set off to soak myself in a tub.

Needless to say soaking in the tub did not work (not on the tape, but it did help me relax a bit).

I am telling you…they put this stuff on with superglue, I just know it! So after convincing my husband to try the polish remover (which took some doing), we got the cotton swabs and set in.

It was slow…very slow….oh my gosh slow! Because it was such a tender area and he had visions of my artery rupturing and squirting blood out everywhere (like we had seen on "Grey's Anatomy" just days or so before). However, we did get it all off (well all the tape, it was days before all the glue was gone, no matter what we did) and soon enough….I was free!

The removal of the staples that lined my face

One of the days I feared most, probably from the beginning, was the day the staples would have to be removed. I knew the staples had to be removed 7-10 days after the surgery, and with *that* amount of time my imagination began to wonder about how bad it could be. Thank goodness for my short attention span now! I knew I would be awake for this part, unlike the surgery, and I had never had anything like it before. Not knowing what lies ahead is always the worst part of anything for me. From time to time my imagination ran wild and for someone who may not be able to visualize very well….I can let my mind run wild with worry. As a young adult I worried so much about every little possibility that I wound up taking a path down "Panic and Anxiety Attack Avenue". My anxiety attacks were so crippling that I became housebound before I decided I had to get well and overcome them for the sake of my two little girls! I had left that lifelong behind me, but recall it clearly enough I knew I did not want to go back there again! Thank goodness getting them removed was not really far away! In the meantime, I would ask my youngest daughter how she felt when she had gotten her's removed and hoped she was right as to what it would be like that for me too.

I was so anxious, I even tried going to the doctor's office a few days early to have them checked. I needed to make sure they were not already ready before the weekend, but no such luck.

So a few days later when the day did come, I was beyond ready and on edge.

My head was still very tender and another stranger was going to be poking at it…. pulling things out of it. Just the thought of letting anyone near my head in this condition (other than my husband) was extremely unnerving, UGH! Let alone having them pull staples out of it! And what probably made it worse was……I had already counted them a million times and there were 35 of them! But what was the alternative? I could not just leave them in there! So off we went….

The waiting room time at my local family physician's office was the worst, it was probably only moments but it seemed like we waited for hours. Once in the exam room, with the nurse practitioner (I was surprised the doctor did not even come in to take a look), removing them only a few quick minutes! One by one she used her little staple puller to pluck at each one like you would pluck your eye brows with tweezers (something else I would not do) but not too bad. All that worry and in moments I again was free! Yeah! BREATHE! The worst, or so I thought, was *finally* over!

Now let's move back towards normal life, slowly!

Over just the first few weeks, since the surgery, the numbness and swelling in my head had decreased greatly, the tenderness in my neck slowly improved, my hair was re-growing over top of the incision (so it was not so ugly or scary) and simple ibuprofen still made the headaches tolerable. Best of all I could be back out of the four walls and among the living and the wonderfully kind people in town again, by mid-February I was back to work!

At this time I worked in the service industry and was finally released to go back part time. I (actually my husband) had been charting and tracking my progress on paper to keep the neurosurgeon up to date on my road to recovery. Hoping all the while that we were exactly where we needed to be. When we shared it with him the end of January, he actually thought I was ahead of where he had expected. I was not on all the medications they had given and expected me to be taking (Yuk!) and still doing well. So he released me to light duty and part time work. Yeah!

Oh, not that being so pampered at home was not great, but being useful and productive is an obsession with me….so off I went. Alternate days with a couple hours each, built quickly up to two 4 hour days and soon into two days in-between those, with 2-3 hour days. I was on a roll…moving back towards normal life again.

This was great…until my progress started leveling off, having short periods of non-noticeable progress. I knew things were surely healing more inside the brain, scalp, and neck…but NOT having progress to log was very hard on me (I am a bean counter...it is what I do and love).

Holding on to hope and a positive attitude grew harder, just as my neurosurgeon had warned…people started seeing me as healed and expecting more. Other than the large scar still healing on my neck, no one would have known what I had just recently lived through. Even I wondered how long it would be before I was back to normal, forgetting the doctors told me that it would be a minimum of 6-8 months to get over the biggest effects. Do you know what 6-8 months feels like? It surely feels a lot longer than it sounds, trust me. While it is 6-8 months, it is also 6-8 months of not being able to be and do all you once did. That, they don't tell you, and your mind doesn't grasp it when they do try to.

     I had already started re-doing the needle work I had messed up earlier and picked up the new Kindle 2 (electronic book) my husband and I bought for ourselves as our anniversary gift. To later take to the beach, he promised. I tried escaping the frustration with needle work, reading a good book, conquering computer games, chatting with friends, and light workouts (we joined the local Y) to get moving. All this, of course, while adding in the new spring sunshine when my husband could get me outside for some good vitamin D healing sessions. And when all else failed, I called the neurosurgeon to explain where I was and for more reassurance that it was still where I should be. Then waited for the next round of signs I was again moving forward with the healing I had yet to do.

The headaches

Getting out into the fresh spring air for some healing vitamin d was a great idea. Or so we thought in the beginning. Unfortunately, we quickly discovered it merely brought on a new form of sudden and extremely painful debilitating headaches with the onset of spring.

And forget gardening (something else I loved about spring), it too brought on similar results but in a different area of my head. Twice my attempts to weed the many flower beds left me nearly laid out amongst the irises waiting for someone to find me, from the pain and weakness that overcame me so quickly.

We quickly decided going outside alone was no longer an option. At least until we figured out what was causing these awful headaches and how to prevent them.

They felt as though someone had hit me in the side of my head with a metal shovel, that my face was peeling off by its self, and left my eye so painful I wanted to rip it out of its socket with my bare hands. It felt as if I was having brain surgery all over again…although this time…I was awake through it all.

Spring had sprung and along with it came terrible pain and sadness. I had such hopes that along with spring, my recovery would grow….and this was a huge set back! Balancing these headaches with the emotional and physical struggle they brought me was nearly *too* much. I could no longer walk, chew gum, and think at the same time and now feeling house bound indefinitely was just too much to bare.

      First we tried sunglasses and a hat whenever I went outside, thinking the sun reflecting off the blind spot (discovered at an earlier appointment) in my vision was at least part of the problem. The blind spot was one side effect of my procedure since the aneurysm was pressing on the optical nerve. Your optical nerve does not liked to be touched and when it is there is immediate damage. At this point there is not a lot known about the damage, as to whether it is permanent or temporary, since there is no real test for that kind of injury…but we'll wait and see.

The hat and sunglasses did help a bit. Glare was definitely part of the issue. However, I still could not go near the gardens or be outside when people were mowing. Even driving to work had now become a challenge with the spring sun and air, people out mowing their lawns, farmers planting their crops, and things blooming everywhere. The added pressure of it all only stirred the struggles I also faced with memory recall. This was when I discovered my new little friend.

Meeting "Mr. Spaz"

A couple months post-surgery, was when I hit one of the next road blocks, the headaches and memory recall issues. This was also when I met "Mr. Spaz". "Mr. Spaz" was the nick name I later gave the lone brain cell I saw in my mind's eye each time I felt my mind panic trying to recall things. At this point, any time I had to recall more than two or three things he became much clearer. I could feel him run *out of control* through my mind each and every time, separately from myself. I could see him clearly...and soon he became my new little friend.
I remember thinking he looked like a character I use to draw in high school or a character that could have existed in a series of books I read to my children when they were small, "Mr. Happy", "Mr. Sneeze", "Mr. Messy" and such, by Roger Hargreaves.

A little blue hairball that looked like he had stuck his wet finger in a light socket, frazzled with all his hair standing on end. All you could see was his little arms and legs sticking out of all that hair and his cute little bowler hat on top his head, of course. Poor little thing was always on the verge, if not in full, panic mode. He was always pleased and proud as punch to be asked to do something, like recall, but clueless as to *how* to do such a thing.

And there in the distance.....my many other brain cells stood just beyond the fog, or just outside of clear view - waiting and wondering when he would get a clue.

They seemed to know, remember, and recall that all he had to do was reach out to any one of them for the information needed. However, not a one of them would reach towards him or give him the single clue of what to do. They seemed bound and determined *he* was the path finder; it would be again his sole job to do.

Poor little guy, panicked in his solitude for months as we played games listing 4 things to choose from for diner, to buy at the grocery, to put on ice cream at night, or anything else we could think of.

Until one day...It worked! He remembered items one through four! And though months later (and now sometimes even years later) it is still a feat that is unreliable, he has learned not to panic or spaz out about it, now knowing that only makes it worse.

I think once he learned he could, that panicking does not help, and that he was not really alone up there in my mind....he grew to realize too how important he really was, with his own special job to do. Like we all come to realize growing up...he learned there is a place and need for everyone no matter what size you are or what the world comes to. I am guessing, like anyone else he just needed to redefine and find his purpose, taking old journeys in new ways.

Four months post-surgery

Four months post-surgery I was still merely working fourteen to fifteen hours a week over four days and could do very little that took too much strength or endurance due to the head pressure. And driving was still limited to keeping the windows up, sunglasses on, and a hat, for coming and going in and out.

I had also come to realize I could not drive, carry on a conversation, and focus on someone else's directions at the same time without almost causing an accident! Not without "Mr. Spaz" (still incapable of handling more than three things) spazing out. Though by this time I did find him funny as well as very frustrating!

He and the headaches were both things I feared I would have to come to live with by this time. However, they were also the things that motivated me to find a remedy, other than to wait until the season changed, to control the pressure. So to help both myself (find relief from the headaches) and

"Mr. Spaz", I scheduled myself yet *another* appointment back with my neurologist.

A few weeks later, there we sat in my neurologist's office…. as he performed those same silly tests over again and then asked me about my concerns in more detail. I told him about the sun and how sunglasses and a hat had helped the eyeball problem, but not the shovel against the brain thing. I told him about my concerns over my memory recall ability (or lack thereof) and even about "Mr. Spaz". I am sure by this point he thought I was just nuts.

He noted everything in his log and then said….. "Well, I guess we need to first get another follow up MRI (with and without contrast, the order later said) for the headaches" and for the recall issue… "I think a neuropsychological evaluation is in order". To which I quickly responded, without much thought…. "Not until after I return from the beach!" and I guess I responded rather quickly, because I almost thought I saw his head spin as he turned and stared at me (LOL).

We had planned a trip to the beach in North Carolina for some time, it was one of our favorite places to go and we were going!

My neurosurgeon had already released me for the trip that my husband had promised me….we were going…and we did! I was over being poked, prodded, and invaded upon. I needed a break! Our wallets needed a break! My husband needed a break! And we were taking it!

It had been a year since we had last gone and taken one of our grandsons (and his parents) to our favorite hot dog stand at the beach...and that was far too long, after all we had been through, it was time we go again! So May 20th we hopped in the already packed car and headed south. Ahh…. finally a vacation! No work, no bills, no responsibilities and best of all … NO DOCTORS WITH PROBING TESTS!

We were just outside of Indiana (where we lived at the time) when I realized for the first time in nearly 6 months…I did not have a headache. Other than the time my oldest sister gave me a Reiki treatment when doctors failed to give me relief themselves.

Suddenly, I was headache free. I did not even have one of those achy ones the ibuprofen usually left me with. However, even in my shock and excitement I waited, thinking surely it was a fluke. So we drove on …for miles…all the way to Durham, North Carolina and with no headache! Not even through the mountains!

The next day, we moved on to Southport, North Carolina and my brother-in-law's place for more family time, more Trolly dogs, and house hunting (something we had been leisurely doing for about two years now, and were boosted with the hope of finding a new way to reinvest our retirement money with the economy as it is these days)….and still NO HEADACHE!

Sunday, with a promise we would take it easy and turn around and come back if any head pain arose…we went boating with my brother-in-law and his wife. We headed for the Cape Fear and out towards the ocean. We were out for nearly 8 hours before returning and still no head pain! It was great! Finally, no more headaches, I was back to normal!

It was not until the return trip back to Indiana reality struck….and the headaches returned. As soon as we reached the mountain area they were back and back with a vengeance! It was now June 1st and by the time I was scheduled for the MRI on June 8th I had not had another day without a headache. It was disappointing to say the least, but by now I had at least figured out *one* of the other headaches causes…..allergies! It had to be sinus pressure from pollen and things that came along with spring. It was spring when my head first started to suffer this kind of pain and it had to be my old allergies creating sinus pressure on my newly surgically sensitive head!

So, off to the MRI I went and anxiously awaited my follow up appointment with my neurologist (yes, two weeks later….ugh) to announce my own findings. Sure enough, the MRI showed not only nothing more than the issues I had had before and the post-operative expectations of a brain that has been through what mine had, but also sinus problems that were probably allergy related. Yeah!

However, that meant more doctors for a solution (UGH again) and we still had not been in for the neuropsychological evaluation. Welcome back to the real world.

On July 10th (seven months post-surgery) I met with the allergist. His staff performed a breath test, took a nasal smear, and sat me in a room to await the doctor.

When he arrived we went over the pre-appointment paperwork sent to me by his staff and then I was prepped for the allergy test it's self.

My entire back was wiped down with alcohol for sanitation. Once prepped small boards containing probably 9 small needles each were dipped in allergens and placed over a section of my back and rocked gently until my entire back had been covered with items to test for. I then sat for about twenty minutes for them to take effect. Given strict instructions not to itch.

After twenty minutes the technician returned to determine the results. She then called in the physician for his input. This is when he declared the test was inconclusive due to the *unique* reaction to the alcohol used to prep my skin. Now, they would need to redo the test in a different way that would not require the use of direct contact with the alcohol. Because apparently I was allergic to the alcohol.

My back was then cleaned and freed of all the markings and labels before she prepared for the new procedure. The alternate route (or procedure) was to inject each allergen in question individually into both my upper and lowers arms. Each shot was then labeled with a number to keep record and another twenty minute wait took place, during which I was asked not to *touch* the areas, "no matter how much they may begin to itch".

The staff again returned twenty minutes later along with the physician and concluded I was reacting to several of the allergens. Those that were reacting were several molds commonly found in the Midwest as well as to a couple of dust mites, commonly found inside the home. I felt immediate (mental) relief. Finally a solution we could find a resolution for that would take the ongoing head pain away again.

However…you know me…."UNIQUE"…..

Before the staff could clean me up and cover the necessary information as to what I could do and how I could avoid the allergens I would react to, I broke out in hives all about my neck (around one of the surgical areas) and rapidly spreading up into my hairline.

The doctor was then called back into the room, took one look, and said "you seem to be allergic to our test"…I merely laughed and said "I told you, I am unique!"

His staff immediately checked my vitals, breathing, and pupils before giving me an oral allergy medication in hopes to stop the reaction quickly. One of the nurses then applied a topical cream to help the itching and was instructed to monitor me frequently. Each few minutes one of the staff would come in ask how I was, look at my neck and check vitals. Quickly the reaction stopped and improved, thankfully, and soon I was sent on my way…with a bag full of new medications, prescriptions and information on how to deal with my allergy driven headaches, of which have yet to do the trick as well as heading south!

By the end of summer

By August, the headaches were still present, but less severe. I still had to wear sunglasses and a hat while outside to cut down glare, though it seemed some of the optical nerve damage had improved (or at least seemed to have leveled off). I continue to practice measuring and exercising it using a make shift eye chart we placed on our dining room wall near the beginning of my recovery process.

We created it in hopes that exercising it (like other parts of the body, post surgeries) would help it recover and since doctors could not dispute it might help…what did we have to loose?

At night (after beginning energy treatments on the affected area) I began to see these extremely white color flashes behind my eyelids. It was much like what I saw during my arteriogram, except now it was merely a series of small dots or stars near the inner corner of my left eye (where the damage had existed post-surgery). I cannot explain it even now and do it justice. However I can tell you that it was beyond any shade of white you have probably ever seen.

When it first started it took me nearly a month before I would return to the eye chart to see what it was doing to my already obstructed vision, for fear of getting my hopes up too high (now a bit leery since the headaches had still been attacking me for so long).

However, one day when I could stand it no longer, I dared to speak to my husband about it out loud and you know how that obligates you to do something. So, of course, we went directly to the chart and were pleasantly surprised that there had been a slight improvement in the area of my peripheral vision since the last time I had checked. What a relief! Even doctors could not contribute the unusual improvement to anything else.

The facial muscle spasms had become less frequent by this point, as well as less intense. The incision area seemed less tender, finally, though I still remained guarded anytime anyone even seemed to come close to it.

My neck incision area was also less intense looking, though still seemed to still scare a child now and then when they noticed it for some time. I found very little luck getting the scar to actually disappear, even with the over-the-counter creams that proclaim to do exactly that. While the area between the scar and my chin remained numb to a large degree and making a very slow journey towards progress towards recovering. Though doctors assured me that over time it would fully return to "normal". There was just no way to know how long it will be.

"Mr. Spaz" remained with me, though his name seemed less and less appropriate by this time. My memory recall was still a bit unreliable, but decreasingly so, which was encouraging. It was nice to once again sense the family of cells reuniting and without hard feelings between them, after their temporary breakdown. Though I knew I was not fully back to where I was.

We never made it to the neuropsychologist, we were too busy with the allergist appointments. Trying to solve those issues became our bigger priority that summer and moving forward. So the neurologist said we could put it off for a time and see what the future held, before we canceled the appointment all together.

As for the allergies, we were still trying to find the right medications that might make it tolerable to continue to live in the Midwest. Adjusting medications and dosages to find just the right blend was not easy as the seasons changed over and over as we tried. However, we remained confident we would get there one day and were encouraged with any small progress along the way.

For a while we got to the beach in North Carolina more often, just because we needed it more and more. The breaks it gave me from the headaches were a huge relief. And since by now we had made a change in our retirement funds by acquiring a new home there...we decided it would be best to make use of it often. We love the area, seeing the other family members more often (including my sister that helped save my life, by sharing her story), and reacquainting with old friends, as well as making new ones. We hoped to find it as loving, supportive, and caring as those we would one day leave behind in the Midwest.

Otherwise, mentally, I was learning to accept the reality that getting back to "Normal Life" would be an ongoing path I would have to choose to greet with more confidence each new day. I was happy to be alive. I took this journey to stay alive and was now recovering and re-discovering the new me that post-brain surgery allows me to be. A path my oldest daughter reminded me WAS the same path I was on before brain surgery. Discovering, as we all do….the new us is someone we re-invent each new day, brain surgery or not. She was right, it was the path I was on before I headed down this road so now it was time for me to get back to life as normal… and continue to do so.

For a while I continued to work part time, gardened when I could (which was seldom) and spent time with family and friends, and began to explore avenues to educate myself on new arts of healing naturally. In hopes to reduce the many medications I now seemed to have to live on as well as reduces the episodes the allergies plagued me with. I worked on receiving my certifications in Reiki and Intuitive Energy Healing. Getting away to our home in North Carolina every chance I got for relief.

When I failed to convince doctors I would find recovery faster if they prescribed me a prescription to move permanently to my new home, I decided to take things into my own hands. Just after my four year anniversary post-surgery I received an offer of employment near our new retirement home. And in no time I found myself packed up and gone. Hoping my husband would also soon find employment here and follow. Unfortunately, he did find new employment but in the same area of our Indiana home as his last. So it would be a long year before his new company would agree to move him south alongside me. However, now ....here he is!

And now here we are...facing my five year review, post-surgery.

Five years post-surgery

Wow, five years post-surgery, are we truly here? Yes, yes we are. This December is my five year anniversary of this journey. What an amazing journey it has been!

I am happy to say, I am still continuing the journey of recovery all these years later. Still taking small steps of progress towards "normal" or at least to the new me crafted from the beginning. Although at times the road has gotten a bit tough, as it does for all those who travel here, here I am still traveling along often filled with renewed hope and wonder.

My taste for gingerbread still remains with me, though tamed just a bit since then. However along with it I found an extreme interest in foods like Key Lime, peach, raspberry, fresh veggies and a few others that escape me right now….maybe still part of my memory recall that remains consistently only unreliable. However, look…I did get past the list of four items that use to stomp me over four years ago.

I seldom see or hear from Mr. Spaz any more, sadly I must admit. Like a new friend made during a tough time, I do miss his sense of humor now and then. However, while I do still have a bit of trouble with reliable short term memory, the peacefulness that acceptance has brought is a bit less destructive then his panic. Sometimes I can recall things thrown at me quickly or items listed over four. Sometimes not. While the inconsistency is a bit stressful at times, the continued growth leads room to hope. Even at my age, now over fifty. Which now that I have turned, doctors tell me "oh don't worry about it, now that you're fifty it's all typical signs of aging and you'll fit right in". "No", I say, that is just unacceptable. Not the turning fifty part, the whole stuffing me into a category of *aging* that makes things like this "normal". Not everyone ages at the same rate and I have had these issues since the surgery not because of my age. And for as long as I see improvement, or reason to hope I will regain my memory losses, the longer I will continue to hope that it will improve with renewed hope.

I do not go to the doctor's office as much at all anymore. Other than the regular checkup that I cannot escape from. Other than the allergist I worked with until recently. My new physician here so far has handled all my medical needs, which are far less than they once were, thankfully. In fact, over this past summer as my anxiety rose at the mere thought of returning to my brain surgeon for the five year review appointment I decided to call his office in hopes of finding out just what the visit would be like. Hoping it would not require yet another angiogram. After what happened the last time, that was the last thing I wanted to go back through.

To my relief the office staff said… "oh no, you will not be required to do another angiogram, merely another CAT scan is all." Yeah! I thought.

Until a moment later she also told me I would need to schedule my follow up appointment with one of the other doctors in the office. My brain surgeon retired (without consulting me) last year. WHAT? Seriously? It is tough walk through this process but now you want to have me reestablish trust with someone who has little more than notes to imagine where I have been? Really?

      I decided that would not be for me. Since all I needed was a CAT scan I thought to myself, my new doctor surely can handle that. Right?

In November I called and scheduled the follow up CAT scan with my new family doctor and showed up for my scheduled appointment at the lab center. Upon my arrival the woman announced she would be administering the dye necessary to get the best results. Until I told her the tale of my experience with the dye from the angiogram. At this time she excused herself to check the records and returned moments later to announce, "Yeah, in your case…I think we will forgo the dye this trip and worry about that if the results show we have something more to worry about." GREAT IDEA!

Thankfully, the CAT scan showed no issues. Instead I got a real view of the titanium clip inside my brain (larger then I imagined) and this funny little thing just inside my scalp I believe was to hold the drain in place post-surgery. It looks like one of those plastic sock holder we once had to hold a pair of socks together, rather them folding them into a ball. Some of you will know what I mean, I am sure.

It was a bit disappointing not to get a true image of the actual aneurysm, but…if it requires the trip I took before with the dye….I will pass gladly.

        As for the scars to my face and neck. They still remain. Though slightly faded and mostly covered by my hair line. Other than the one on my neck…no one seems to notice nearly as much. I still rub them often, as advised by doctors then, to reduce scar tissue. Though it only makes the side of my head pop, which grosses people out.

The numbness in my chin and neck caused by the incision there to hold the artery still during surgery, is still progressing slowly as well. I can feel much more of the area then immediately following surgery. However, there is still a small area that has some numbness at certain depths that continues to improve, very slowly. Though as long as there is improvement I am happy.

As for my vision loss post-surgery, doctors are still not sure how I recovered that small amount of loss early on. Though testing proves it is still there, I have gained little to no more. I however, still credit the recovery to the work I did to keep the area exercised and stimulated with healing energy. Both of which I no longer do regularly but toy with from time to time. The little loss I do have resides just inside the left eyes field of vision. Where if you close your right eye and use only your left, you would see your nose. For me, mine is there, just very distorted or blurry. So I count myself blessed and choose not to *focus* on it.

The terrible headaches continue to approach though less often over time. Though I can experience them if I over exert, get over heated, or expose myself to my allergy triggers. The allergies being the toughest over all. Until moving here it took a lot of testing, retesting, experimenting and re-experimenting with one medication (or combination of many) before doctors could find the right blend for each cause of each individual kind of headache/allergy.

However, the move south was definitely the biggest and best prescription yet. If I do say so myself.

For the most part these days I can keep the headaches at bay and am doing so with a lot less medication. The medications that in time only made me extremely tired or began offering other negative side effects.

The biggest hurtle to stopping the headaches began with the discovery and diagnosis of an allergy to cleaning chemicals. Before my move south, while at work one day, I spent some time helping to clean. Shortly after beginning I could feel the room grow stuffy, found it difficult to breath and became very weak. In a split second I was laying on a table nearby feeling myself breath but getting little to no air. It was not until a fellow employee came over to take my hands in prayer that I began to feel even the slightest bit better. A short time later, my husband arrived to take me to the hospital. However, once outside I immediately began to feel better. And by the time we arrived doctors were amazed at how fast anaphylaxis shock had taken over due to an unknown allergy.

When I returned to work, my boss issued me one order, "don't you ever do that again, I have never seen a live person turn that shade of gray, and never want to see it again!" Me either!

However, though not as severe I would do so nearly four more times before doctors committed my allergy to being to *ANY form of cleaning chemical*. From hand sanitizers, rubbing alcohol, to scrubs and bleach, window cleaners and all. Each brings it's on strength of headache, breathing problems and now levels of hives as well. And while everyone says "I wish I had that issue, so I wouldn't have to clean my house" trust me if they did….they would truly hope they did not! It is not the fun it seems it would be.

It took more doctor visits, more poking and prodding and more testing as well as even more medications to merely *hope* to give me some reaction or *escape* time when exposed. There is no magic medical cure. So my job became finding other alternatives or learn to try to learn live with it.

For me *living* with it was the main key focus, since every time I turned around someone was inadvertently trying to kill me with one cleaning chemical or another. You have no idea how many people you cross paths with in a single day that expose you to some cleaning chemical or another until you are this allergic to them. Gas stations, restaurants, grocery or other shopping centers, and most of all hospitals and doctor's offices. Someone is constantly hand sanitizing their hands or a cart, wipes a counter top or cleans off a table for you (or nearby), someone mops a floor in the area, cleans trays or cleans a window or glass door (the list goes on and on).

It is exhausting to try to stay clear of them all, especially when your sense of smell is so hyper sensitive but can no longer speak to your brain or no longer speaks to it in a language it understands. The one thing doctors are yet sure of in my case. Is it that my brain no longer hears what my sense of smell tells it? Or is it that it can no longer get the message through to it? Or is it that the message is going through but no longer translates properly. Who knows?

So for the last couple of years I have sung to myself "Oxygen good, everything else BAD" hoping in time the mantra would teach my brain new tricks to understanding *chemicals are not friends*.

For the first couple years I carried an inhaler, an EpiPen, extra allergy medications, ibuprofen, and another pain reliever (because sometimes one worked, sometimes the other) and a mess more tricks to try to stay alive. Which I must admit, I still carry just encase. However seldom pull out any more. Thanks to a young woman that works at my new favorite store in Wilmington (a town nearby).

Once diagnosed with the cleaning chemical allergy and doctors said there was no medication or cure, I set myself on a trek to find something that would help. Either something that would help me live with it easier (and without taking drugs) or something that would completely illuminate it all together. You see, my problem was not just that I could not use them or be exposed to them, but that they were constantly trying to snuff out my very life each time I was. This had to stop! I was not afraid of death, merely did not feel ready to go and unwilling to go that way. Especially now that I was back living at the beach!

So after many trips to the hospital with near misses, I set out to find my own answers. I researched on the internet, I asked friends and family, I spoke to total strangers, asked every doctor I met, and talked to every medical staff person who came close. Medically people especially love a medical mystery. They are sure they have heard them all…so tell them something new and they are hooked. Though unfortunately for me, they offered little solutions.

I tried Reiki, Intuitive Energy Healing, Yoga, Meditation/Mantras, Faster EFT, visiting a Shamin, tested crystal and light therapy, and finally ventured into the world of essential oils. Each bring stress reduction, a more peaceful mind, healing other issues less important at the time, or just feeling great in and of themselves.

But none bringing a solution until I tried the essential oils.

It started with frankincense. An oil given to me by the Shamin I visited. While using it, it did not help with the chemical allergy but did feel refreshing and revitalizing to my face and did affect my breathing to some degree. So after purchasing a small bottle I began to wash my face each morning with a small amount of it and found myself with yet another tool to enhance the start of each new day. When I ran low, I ventured into a nearby essential oil store someone had mentioned to me in down town Wilmington. The store is called "Down to Earth" and is located on Front Street on the back side of Wilmington's Cotton Exchange. The place is filled with a variety of essential oils, fragrance oils, incense, and other things that come in forms like lotions, sprays, soaps, oils and salts. They have oils in small bottles, dropper bottles, and diffusers. And to top it all off they have a great staff that is not only eager to help but are also very informative.

No this is not a commercial for "Down to Earth". However, believe me when you find something, someone, or some place that holds the answer to saving your life….well I hope you understand…they surely deserve the plug.

Anyway….where was I…..

Oh yes, the employee with the magic key. While visiting the store for the first or second time I came across an employee who was eager to help me find just what I might need. When she approached with such confidence I decided I would challenger her with my plight. I told her about my chemical allergy and the helplessness it left me with. When she began to give me her idea with a bit less confidence it would be sure to work, I told her "hey, I am desperate, at this point...I will try anything once". So she sent me home with a blend of essential oils they call "Burglar Blend". An essential oil blend of such things as Eucalyptus, Rosemary, Cinnamon, Clove, Lemon, and Lavender, I believe.

At first use the blend gave me terrible headaches, though did seem to open my airways a bit. So upon my return to the store I told her so. This is when she suggested that the blend might be too strong for my hypersensitive sense of smell. Her suggestion was to blend the mixture with equal parts Polysorbate 20, place the new mixture in a mister bottle and mist about my neck and wrist areas as needed.

The next few times I was exposed to cleaning chemicals and began to feel their affects I used the new misting blend. Immediately I felt relief both in my breathing and in my own peace of mind. Thank goodness! Finally! Something in the form of success. Over the next few weeks I continued to use the product any time I had difficulties being near cleaning agents. The little mister bottle went with me everywhere! I told everyone what it was, where I got it and all about the young woman who has now helped save my life.

However, the story does not end there. For you see….now a few months later….and I have noticed that not only does the mixture help support my breathing system in times of trouble but has begun to speak the language my sense of smell needs to get my brain to listen and head the warning when chemicals are near. The first few moments someone begins to expose me with a cleaning agent within a few feet, I now can smell the agent, detect where it is coming from and merely have to move approximately three feet away (rather than run for my life, as I once did) to remain safe. The blend of oils misted upon my skin has allowed me to change the way my sense of smell speaks to my brain and allows my brain to speak to the rest of me and say "Hey…look….someone is cleaning over there, might want to adjust your space and breathing technique if you want to live longer".

So as you might guess, I have not only returned to "Down to Earth" essential oil store many times and complimented the young woman, but have continued to send more and more customers her way. Forever grateful for the freedom to live amongst others once again, dinning out, shopping, going for routine checkups and visiting those family members obsessed with cleaning (who have not yet gone *GREEN* like my daughter, Libbie, and I).

You do not need all those harsh chemicals to clean your home prompted by stores, commercials and sales gimmicks. Simple vinegar, lemon juice, sea salt and such can do the tricks quite nicely. You would be amazed. Even on weeds, just a half cup of sea salt, a spray bottle full of vinegar and a large squirt of dish soap on a hot summer morning kills grass and weeds from any walk way or flower bed, without harmful pesticides. And for your laundry, Libbie taught me, a bit of Fels Naptha soap, Arm and Hammer Super Washing Soda and Borax mixed in to hot water then poured into a large bucket filled with more water, set over night…and presto you have 10 gallons of homemade laundry soap that cleans well and will not irritate even the most sensitive skin. You can even add an essential oil to create your own scent if you would like.

Try it!

The reflection collection:

The following pages are some of the many writings I wrote early on post-surgery. Something yet again….I did before and continue to do today. I hope you enjoy my ramblings.

Today...

Today is yet a day gone by, tomorrow.

But tomorrow is a day we greet with hope,

anticipation and a bundle full of dreams.

He Stood By Me

For years my now husband and I have been friends
Until years later life gave us
The opportunity..
To become more
Leading us to fall in love
And married,
And he stood by me.

About three years later doctors told him
Your wife has a brain aneurysm
She needs tests and appointments
And through it all
And he stood by me.

Through every appointment
Through every announcement
Through every test
Through every medication
Through every reaction, followed by more medication
Through every recovery period (none of which were pretty)
He still stood by me.

Hours on the table

With someone else's hands in my brain
Helpless to do anything…alone
He still stood by me.

Facing me hours later
With my head split open and swollen
Black and blue with staples tracing my hairline
He still stood by me.

Days of cleaning my incisions
Weeks of giving me pain med timely
Months of being there at my beck and call
(again not always pretty)
He still stood by me.

Months of medical bills
Months out of work (for recovery)
Months of pain he could do little to take away
Months more of follow up appointments
Months more of tests
And yet he still stood by me.

With love like no other, my husband....Will
Still stands by me.

Memories Are Left Behind

Memories are always left behind us
In everything we do.
Good or bad, we remember
Every little move,
Separated as into boxes
We treat them all with care.
Trying to hang on to the good
Setting the bad free, into the air.
Often we are reminded of both
the good and bad
And the pain returns along with them
Leaving us feeling sad
Hoping that someday
There'll be one to replace the last
To carry it far away.

Clay

I believe my being began...
Much like being a glob of clay
And whether you believe in a higher power
That created me
Or...
In science that says the genes of two
Joined to become one....
I came to be that glob of clay.

Clay placed on a wheel
Much like clay placed on a potter's wheel
I was placed however so
On the wheel of life
When my life began.
Over the years life has molded me
Into who and what I am
Ever changing what I appear to be.
Each person and life experience molding
A piece of me into something new.
Leaving me forever changed with each spin
Forever inspired to do more and be more.

My beauty is in the eye of the beholder
Who sees in me...

What service my presence serves them.
With each glance I am renewed

With each turn I reflect difference
And with each new experience
I change...like molded clay.
Forever changing
Becoming more
As long as my heart does not harden
With the onset of each new day.

Forget not to soften and sooth me
With the bit of support I require
To remain soft and pliable in your hands
To be all that I was created in my depth...to be.

Welcome

Welcome to life's journey

Where you will have no control

Over the path in which you live

But merely be an observer of the

Changes your mind and body go through

Thank goodness you've been given a soul

To which faith

May pour through

And give you peace

Like no other!

The Conversation Dance

What happened to take a deep breath..
Count to ten?
Is it only for those who are angry?
I think not.
Counting to ten...
Should be for when the drama begins
And distracts you from sharing who you are
With those who most need to see you.
When the drama starts,
Do we stop and ask someone...
would you like to talk?
Or I need to talk....can you listen to me right now?
Yet when the music starts we ask....
Would you like to dance?

The Drama

Something happens (the drama) in
someone's life
That stirs thoughts, feelings and emotions.
It's human nature verses life.
And at some point..
They find they need to be seen, recognized
and understood.

It isn't always about being right or wrong,
It is often about being noticed, valued...
For who they are in that moment.

We are what we think,
We are what we feel,
We are what we perceive,
We are!

But we are not always what we paint
Or what others perceive us to be.
Something we often forget.
If we could look at another
With wonderment.
As if we don't know them
And ask....
Who are you today?

That would be most the key,

To unlocking all the drama…
And truly be able to see
Who each of us mean to be.

For Years….

For years we learned to work
To accomplish all we wanted
Now.....
How long will it take to learn to sacrifice?
All we don't really need...
For what we had and should have valued all along?
The faster we learned this lesson....
The faster we will again move on.
Except this time...
We might just find..
The true happiness we always deserved to begin with.
And appreciate it as much as we always should have.

Brain aneurysm recovery..... A journey of discovery

What they don't tell you.....is what recovery will be like, really.

Because in each person it is different and listing it out....probably impossible.

Too bad more of us who have gone through and survived it….. do not publish more for those who will soon have to. A list of possible issues, thoughts, experiences would be helpful to those who follow....to know some of the things they think and go through might be okay, if not normal.

It is a long and winding road of unknown symptoms and experiences.

A slow process that takes days, months, and now they tell me years...depending on what you are waiting to change back to normal… or the hope of it. And while you go through it...you must remind yourself....but I survived!

I am blessed to be alive.

You must see it as a new adventure.....and face that path of discovery with wonder for your new life.

Once the staples are out, the swelling goes down, you can focus on things longer than a moment here and there, and SOME strength and energy comes back.....and you get those first real ....back to normal life feelings....there is:

The questions of what can I do, when, for how long, and how will that change from day to day?

There are sleep issues, because you haven't done enough to be tired, the....I have an aching pain all the time in my head...but at least it isn't pain like it has been.

The questions about when will my memory return to normal, because your short term or more is affected, lingers or comes up repeatedly.

The numbness in your head (and your neck ...if they also had to cut through to the artery) that hasn't stopped or slowed its progress...and wondering how long that will last.

The tingling and needle poking shooting pains or burning...off and on and off and on........

The new taste changes....smell changes.....vision changes....all wavering to confuse you as to what will be the new normal to adjust to.

You really are a new person with a new chance...but getting to know yourself is difficult...because for now, and for a while, you are in a state of flux....and no one knows how long it will last.

Some last moments...some days....some weeks...till you think okay...this one is set now in who I am....till one day....it changes again! And there is yet another path to the new you created...or modified for a while again.

Never have I felt in such an uncontrolled state of flux...maybe puberty? LOL

At this stage...one day the numb areas are larger....next smaller...next larger again.

You can talk faster....and listen faster...but then....someone says something at just the right speed and you have lost that third item they mentioned. You know you heard it...you know it is in there....but can you recall it? NOPE Not till they repeat it...and then...OH YES, I heard that!

Once the hair has grown back and you can begin to live life close to what it was........others wonder (as you do yourself) how long this recovery will go on? When and why things are not back to normal? You look fine, so......you can see why they begin to forget....and wish for the days you can.

Doctors say...it's a process. But no one tells you how you will think or feel about the process. And as hard as some try to understand....Until they wear the shoe, you hope they never do....they don't and you know it.

All you want is to get back to normal, it's what everyone wants. But no one can tell you what normal is or will be...nor can you tell them. Other than...your alive...and well and moving on.
Some have depression, confusion beyond belief, blindness, and so much more. I am fortunate, I don't have those.....and I am still alive! My side effects of the journey I took

and the path I am on....is much better then some. And I am grateful for that!

But we each have those of our own we still have to learn to cope and adjust through.

And I think if we journal them....it could help not only ourselves but maybe someone new too.

If doctors could ask....what is one trait we should look for when reviewing candidates for this procedure…. I would tell them PATIENCE beyond belief. That...and faith. Even a sense of humor would be nice.

This has truly been a test of patience, patience pushed to the ultimate level.

To face a journey of unknown discovery into a world few seem to really know or understand much about. One in which intrigues me now for reasons beyond my own. Where will it lead me..........who knows..........but definitely renews my hope, perception, and views.

If you have wondered down this path....let me know what has happened to you. Maybe we can inspire each other and create something new.

What you don't know…

Who said what you don't know won't hurt you?

Whoever did....never had or knew they had a brain aneurysm!
And those of us who have...hope they never do.

Some of us have no signs or symptoms.
No warnings
And yet are blessed enough to have something aid medical specialist in finding it.

I was that blessed and more.

Mine was found before it ruptured and caused more damage or my own death.

In a few short weeks, I went from being annoyed with increasing hearing loss (which at my age...might be somewhat uncommon, but isn't really rare) to going from doctor to doctor, having test to procedure and finally....a procedure that hopefully means I will never have to go down this path again...at least not with this aneurysm!

This is just an example of things that could be out of your control. And should focus you on living each day as if it is your last or best moment.

Appreciate all those things in your life and all those who you love.

Live each moment to its fullest.
And allow yourself to think things through the best you can....but don't let the stress of issues rob you of living the life you have while you have it.

Your issue might be a hiding aneurysm...it might be something else. Or you may be blessed in some other way. You may have warning signs....or you might not.

I pray you are fortunate, blessed or whatever you call it....to live beyond what road blocks you.

I am grateful for the opportunity to reach beyond mine into the recovery period I have now.

And for all those that have supported and seen me through it.
Only hoping I have been an inspiration to all of you...to live life as it's meant for you.

And know....what you don't know ....could hurt you....but shouldn't be permitted to stop you from being the best you.

Back to basics......friends!

In these tough times....it is time we all remember what we truly need in life and learn to be happy with knowing we still have at least that.

If you look back in life and recall when life seemed much simpler and fun and etc.....is it not a time when you could......

Get through the school day, hanging out with your friends, share life experiences (ups and downs) over a beer, wine (or whatever your "item" of choice was) and know that each day ended only to be followed knowing you would see them again tomorrow and do it all over?

Then isn't getting back to the basics about being able to get up each new day, doing what you must, so that you can reconnect with old friends (and/or making new ones) over a beer, wine (or whatever)...accept this time legally...... sharing life experiences (ups and downs) and know that each day will be followed knowing they are still there to do it all over again?

View points

Everything looks different from each view point you open your mind to.
With the insight of others.....you are given options not previously open to your awareness.

And in considering them....you can become a more informed, more improved you!

If it weren't for opening to the view point of others:

Oldest children would resent their younger siblings for being burdened with the pressures of being responsible for being the role model for their futures.

Middle children would be forever lost and feeling not as special and that first child that gave their parent those first WOW's they never knew before.

And the youngest children would never learn that they are heard, are noticed and are as important as the others, in their own way.

If it weren't for opening to the view point of others:

Children would never get over feeling to blame for one parents leaving. Never realizing it had nothing to do with you. It was all about them and how they viewed things within themselves.

If it weren't for opening to the views of others:

We would never find our own peace within ourselves that we can live with, to be truly happy. If it weren't for opening to the views of others:
We would be so cut short of all the possibilities that reside outside our own life experiences.

And so much more.......................

Life Comes Alive

Like a sunrise over the ocean
The feelings came alive
Slowly from within me
Building a warmer stronger glow
As time passed
Bringing with it
The sights and sounds
Of life coming more alive
With the song only birds know
The music only lovers hear
Sets my soul gliding ever slowly
With a rhythm I've only come to know
The gracefulness of
The roaring of the rolling waves
Crashing into shore
Bringing with it bits and pieces
Of what there is yet to explore
Taking back out with it
Only the dirt left behind
From days gone past.

Collections

Whether it's a box, jar, book or board......
Every home should have one.....
Placed in it's center (the heart)....As a focal point.

One in which....
All those that pass by.....
Would place their positive, most pleasant thoughts, pictures or memories.

Those we tinker with and keep inside ourselves.
And those we shared with friends and loved ones.
Of fun....kindness......or support and encouragement.

A place where all may go to reflect.....
Whenever we (or others) need them most.
A laugh, hug, or cheering on!

Reminders of what is most valuable....
Memories of days gone by...
And times that lie ahead...
Just waiting ....
For those that pass by.

In Closing:

I remain forever thankful to have my loving supportive husband, family, and many (old and new) friends who remained by my side. Thankful for the opportunity to learn about the value of true friendship traveling this path has taught me through all of you.

And while I am no longer living amongst the small town of Batesville Indiana, I must say too all of you….. you are all included in that group I am forever grateful for. I have been so blessed to have each and every one of you take your step along my path only to make it sparkle a bit more. It is my hope moving forward that I too may inspire others as you have all inspired me in some way.

To my readers, I hope that in reading this you have found the information and knowledge you sought to help support you in your journey ahead either in your life or to pass along to others in theirs. At very least that through love, meditation, and laughter you can make your life or the life of someone near you easier to travel through. It is also my hope that when modern medicine seems to not have all the answers each of you will consider exploring the avenues of natural healing in the arts such as: Reiki, Intuitive Energy Healing, Healing Hands or Healing Touch, Essential Oils, Faster EFT, Chakra Balancing, Yoga, and Mantras/Meditations. You just might be surprised at how many answers to your unresolved heath mysteries you can find and illuminate here. Just like my gaining control over the headaches and life threatening chemical allergies that have been a direct result of surgery. Not only may you find possible remedies and cures in these arts, but best of all you *will* find....***Peace of mind***, just when you need it most!

Thank you for your support,

Mary Ann Windham

Author and Survivor

Also enjoy reading my books:

Inspiration", *a book of poetry finally put in book form due to the inspiration of my mother Patricia.*

And

"Her Story", *for some ghostly adventures with new and old friends. As well as insight on our new home town area back down South.*

Dedication:

Of course to begin I wish to thank my loving husband, Will Windham. Whose love, support, dedication and efforts (and great note taking) far surpassed my hopes and dreams. Truly he set the bar high for any medical advocate/partner. I am forever grateful and truly blessed for having had him brought into this role in life.

To my children, Maurie, Libbie and Jessie, I have always felt so blessed to have been assigned role of your "mother", in this life time. I will never be able to tell each of you enough how very much I love each of you, here. I am so grateful for the many days to come we will still have moving forward through our journey to grow and teach one another all there is. I look forward to the moments moving forward with each of you in new ways and sharing them with the blessings you continue to bring into our lives through our grandchildren. Devan, Dyllan, Kaleb, Gavin, Skyler, Braden, Baylee, and the next one now on the way!

We are both ever so grateful for the many friend and towns people of Batesville, Indiana that serve and visit the local McDonalds. The love, encouragement and support for both myself and husband could have never been foreseen or matched. Bless you all! Including Molly and Dan for those awesome gingerbread cookies!

We also want to thank many of the physicians and their staff who supported us along our way.

Like (but not limited to):

<u>Dr Micheal Pritz</u>, whose excellent work lies mostly inside my head. And <u>Dr Tejada</u>, who also lent his support there. Both serving (then) at IU Medical Center, Indianapolis, Indiana.

And <u>Dr Christopher Stevens</u>, the awesome ENT in Batesville, Indiana who took my healthcare so serious he offered his personal phone number to the Neurologist's office that wanted me to wait months to be seen in the very beginning.

And <u>Dr Robert Petry</u>, my allergist who helped diagnose most of my many *allergies that came as a result of the journey...before they took my life.*

And once again I must thank those many natural healers who have added support to our post-surgery recovery period. Those that began with my oldest sister Debbie and continued with too many others to list since.

May all of your lives be sprinkled with the magical blessings of the pixie dust, love, and light from Spirit far beyond your imaginations as well, forever more.

www.ingramcontent.com/pod-product-compliance
Lightning Source LLC
Chambersburg PA
CBHW051719170526
45167CB00002B/726